Morgan J. Vincent

Muscle Matters

Building Muscle to Reverse Aging & Unlock Longevity

Contents

1.

2.

3.

4.

5.

6.

7.

8.

9.

10.

Introduction

Strength is the Key to Longevity

"If your muscles are strong, you live better." Dr. Gabrielle Lyon

We hear about the Fountain of Youth, and everyone is trying to sell us this cream, vitamin, pill, drink, procedure, or 'cure' that will unlock the secret of youth for us.

Over the past decade, consumer spending on products and services combating aging and enhancing longevity has grown significantly. In 2023, the global anti-aging market was valued at approximately $47 billion and is projected to reach nearly $80 billion by 2032, reflecting a compound annual growth rate (CAGR) of around 6%.

The fitness, aesthetic, and aging market contains a wide array of products and services, including skincare treatments, hair care solutions, cosmetic procedures, dental care, dietary supplements, and fitness programs, all designed to mitigate the visible effects of aging. The primary focus has been on skin and hair treatments, with an expanding emphasis on cosmetic procedures and wellness.

Consumer investment in anti-aging and longevity-enhancing products has grown considerably over the past decade, reaching tens of billions of dollars globally. However, this spending constitutes a relatively small percentage of total healthcare expenditures.

What if you discovered that most of this money is completely wasted? What if there was a way to effectively increase your longevity without spending hundreds or thousands of dollars individually? The possibility is there, right in front of us, and easily obtained by most people living on this earth today. Look, we are all going to die one day. I'm not promising that you'll live forever, just that you can live a longer, healthier quality of life if you make a few changes.

I'm one of those people, the ones constantly looking for new ideas, regimens, or supplements that will help me live a healthier life and improve the damage I've done to my body over the years. You should see my vitamin cabinet! I even work in an industry that supports looking youthful and have spent 20 years learning, training, and practicing my findings. I often wondered why there was not more research on <u>true longevity</u>, the kind that doesn't come in a bottle. To my immense joy, it is happening, or at least coming to light more readily than in the past. Many thought leaders are shedding light on just this concept of true longevity.

One often overlooked yet critical factor is strength in the quest for a longer, healthier life. While many focus on diets, supplements, or anti-aging skincare, research consistently highlights the role of muscle mass and strength in extending lifespan and improving quality of life. Strength is the actual key to true longevity.Building and maintaining muscle goes beyond aesthetics—it's a cornerstone of overall health, vitality, and resilience as we age. Strength is not merely a sign of youth; it's an investment in longevity. Let's dive in and learn more about how muscle mass affects longevity.

The Connection Between Muscle Building and Reversing Aging

Muscle building directly counteracts several key aspects of aging, including the gradual loss of muscle mass and strength, known as sarcopenia. Studies show that adults can lose up to 8% of muscle mass per decade starting in their 30s, and this rate accelerates after age 60 and for women after menopause. This decline has been linked to reduced mobility, higher risks of falls and fractures, and chronic diseases such as diabetes and cardiovascular issues. Regular strength training can reverse these effects by improving muscle mass, bone density, and metabolic health.

Strength training triggers the release of beneficial hormones like growth hormone and insulin-like growth factor (IGF-1), which aid tissue repair and cellular health. It also enhances mitochondrial function, improving energy levels and delaying cellular aging. These combined effects help combat both the visible and underlying markers of aging, emphasizing the essential role of strength in achieving a longer, healthier life.

Why Maintaining and Building Muscle Is Essential at Any Stage of Life

You may think of strength training as a practice primarily for athletes or the young, but its benefits extend to people of all ages and walks of life. For older adults, maintaining muscle mass helps preserve independence and reduces the likelihood of falls and injuries. Strength training also improves balance, coordination, and joint health, which declines with age. Individuals can enhance their physical capabilities by building muscle at any stage and slowing down age-related weakening.

For younger individuals, making muscle building a priority early in life lays the foundation for long-term health. Starting strength training early helps establish habits that prevent premature aging and chronic illnesses later in life. Beyond the physical benefits, building muscle has profound psychological impacts by releasing dopamine and endorphins for overall feeling good, improving confidence, and reducing anxiety. No matter the age or starting point, it's never too late—or too early—to prioritize muscle strength. Muscles have memory and the ability to regain muscle mass and strength more quickly after a break from training. Who wouldn't want to build muscle while they are young to keep waking it up?

Many people are hesitant to embrace this practice later in life. They think of strength training or lifting weights as a teenager or young adult sport. Strength training is one of the most effective tools for improving health across all demographics. Research indicates that older adults can achieve significant muscle mass and strength gains with proper training, even into their 80s and beyond. Starting late is far better than not starting at all, as the body can adapt and improve.

Misconceptions are common with strength training, and many think they require intense, high-impact workouts. Definitely not. Effective strength-building can be achieved through moderate, low-impact exercises tailored to your individual needs and abilities. Resistance bands, bodyweight exercises, and light weights, including kettlebells, are accessible options that yield impressive results over time. Strength training is age-friendly and the practice of it can be transformative for enhancing longevity and overall health.

I

Part One

1

The Science of Muscle and Aging

Let's be honest with ourselves: aging is an inevitable process. We are all aging every minute of every day, year after year, but the condition of our muscle mass can influence how we age. Far from just being a cosmetic concern, muscle health is pivotal in determining longevity and overall well-being. This chapter delves into the science behind muscle and aging, exploring how muscle mass impacts health, the physiological changes that occur with age, and why muscle is often called the "organ of longevity."

How Aging Affects Muscle Mass and Overall Health (Sarcopenia Explained)

One of the most significant effects of aging on the body is the loss of muscle mass and strength, which is a condition known as sarcopenia. This gradual decline typically begins in the 30s, yes, in your 30s! with an estimated 3–5% loss of muscle mass per decade. By the time you reach your 70s, you may have lost up to 50% of your peak muscle mass if no interventions are undertaken. Sarcopenia isn't just about weaker muscles or reduced muscle mass; it has a ripple effect on overall health, increasing the risk of falls, fractures, mobility limitations, dependency, and even immune health.

Sarcopenia occurs due to a combination of factors, including hormonal changes, reduced physical activity, and a decrease in the body's ability to synthesize protein. Sarcopenia leads to diminished strength and endurance, which impairs the body's ability to perform everyday tasks and compromises independence. Resistance & strength training, along with adequate *absorbable* protein in,take can significantly slow or even reverse sarcopenia, emphasizing the importance of proactive muscle maintenance throughout life.

How Does Muscle Impact Metabolic Health, Bone Density, and Disease Prevention?

Muscle is more than a mechanism for movement; it is integral to metabolic health and disease prevention. Muscles act as a primary reservoir for glucose and, therefore play a critical role in regulating blood sugar levels and preventing insulin resistance—a key factor in developing type 2 diabetes. Additionally, maintaining or increasing muscle mass supports a higher resting metabolic rate, improving weight management and reducing the risk of obesity-related diseases.

Dr. Gabrielle Lyon [2], a functional medicine practitioner and board-certified family medicine physician, works to shift "the focus away from reactively quantifying and treating disease to proactively quantifying and optimizing your health by focusing on the biggest organ in your body: skeletal muscle." She is famously known for her take, "We aren't over fat; we are just under-muscled." Because we have "an unhealthy muscle problem which is leading to diseases and chronic aging." [3]

Beyond metabolism, muscle contributes to bone density by exerting mechanical stress on bones during movement. This stress stimulates bone remodeling and strengthens skeletal structures, reducing the risk of osteoporosis and fractures. Muscle health is linked to cardiovascular function, as stronger muscles enhance circulation and reduce strain on the heart. If we can prevent chronic conditions such as diabetes, heart disease, and osteoporosis, muscle is a cornerstone for long-term health and resilience.

We have all sorts of excuses why we can't strength train or exercise: life is too busy, the kids have after-school activities, I'm exhausted from work, I've got to clean the house, it's dinner time, it's too cold/hot outside, etc. One of my favorite quotes is, "Don't be upset about the results you didn't get with the work you didn't do" by Dr. Eric Cobb. He's right. No excuse you can come up with will replace the results you could have if you take this information seriously and do something with it.

Why Muscle Is the "Organ of Longevity"

Years ago, I was taught that the largest organ in the body is the skin. But as time marches on, we find that muscle is becoming the largest organ, and it has earned the moniker "organ of longevity" because its benefits extend far beyond physical strength. It functions as an endocrine organ, releasing myokines—signaling molecules communicating with other tissues and organs. Myokines have anti-inflammatory and protective effects on the brain, heart, and immune system, highlighting muscle's systemic influence on health. Myokines play a crucial role in reducing inflammation, which is a significant contributor to aging and age-related diseases.

Muscle health is closely associated with mortality rates. Studies have shown that higher muscle mass and strength are linked to lower risks of all-cause mortality, independent of body fat levels. By supporting mobility, balance, metabolic health, and systemic resilience, muscle becomes essential in extending both lifespan and health span—the years spent in good health. Physical strength is the foundation of longevity.

2

Building Muscle, Reversing Aging

Strength training is more than just lifting weights; it is a method to reversing many signs of aging and improving overall health that is backed by science and numerous studies. Building muscle can impact aging by stimulating cellular regeneration, reducing inflammation, and enhancing insulin sensitivity in our bodies. And let's be honest, we feel better after a great workout, which lasts for hours, if not longer. Let's explore how strength training supports healthy aging, from preventing chronic diseases to reclaiming energy, mobility, and independence.

Impact Cellular Regeneration, Reduce Inflammation, and Promote Healthy Aging

At the cellular level, strength training has a rejuvenating effect on the body. While we perform resistance exercises, our muscle fibers undergo microscopic damage, which triggers a repair function that strengthens and regenerates the tissue. This process activates satellite cells—specialized stem cells responsible for muscle growth and regeneration. Over time, these activities enhance our muscle strength and cellular vitality, lining us up to enjoy healthier aging.

Strength training also significantly reduces chronic inflammation, a hallmark of aging and many age-related diseases. Regular exercise stimulates the release of myokines, anti-inflammatory proteins secreted by muscles. They help regulate immune responses and reduce dangerous inflammation. Inflammation is something to avoid agressively. It accelerates cellular aging and contributes to conditions like arthritis, heart disease, and cognitive decline. Strength training also boosts mitochondrial function, improving energy production and combating oxidative stress, further promoting cellular health and longevity. There are even more benefits of strength training that we may not be able to record but we recognize in our bodies over time.

The Benefits of Muscle Building for Improving Insulin Sensitivity and Reducing Chronic Disease Risks

Building muscle profoundly impacts metabolic health, particularly in enhancing insulin sensitivity. Muscles act as a glucose reservoir, and strength training increases their ability to take up and utilize glucose efficiently. This improved glucose metabolism reduces insulin resistance, which is a key driver of type 2 diabetes and metabolic syndrome. In fact, individuals who engage in regular strength training are significantly less likely to develop diabetes compared to their sedentary peers.

Beyond metabolic health, muscle building lowers the risk of other chronic diseases. By reducing dangerous visceral fat that surrounds our organs, improving cardiovascular function, and enhancing bone density, strength training reduces risks associated with obesity, heart disease, and osteoporosis. Stronger muscles lessen the likelihood of falls and related injuries, which are a leading cause of disability and mortality among older adults. Together, these benefits highlight muscle building as a powerful preventative tool for long-term health.

Reclaiming Energy, Mobility, and Independence Through Strength Training

One of the most immediate and noticeable benefits of strength training is restoring energy levels. As we age, any source of natural energy is welcome by me! Regular resistance exercise improves circulation, boosts endorphin production, and enhances mitochondrial efficiency, all contributing to increased vitality. This newfound energy extends beyond the gym, empowers us to engage more fully in daily activities and hobbieswe.

Strengthening muscles, tendons, and ligaments enhance stability and balance, reducing the risk of falls. Improved joint health and flexibility make everyday movements—like climbing stairs, carrying groceries, or playing with grandchildren—easier and pain-free. For many, this renewed mobility translates into greater autonomy and quality of life. It's never too late to start reclaiming strength and independence. Start today if you do not already have a system in place. Strength training is not only a path to building muscle but also a gateway to reversing the physical and systemic effects of aging. Strength training redefines what aging looks and feels like through its impact on cellular regeneration, chronic disease prevention, and physical capability.

3

Creating a Sustainable Strength Training Plan

The key to long-term success with strength training lies in sustainability. Creating a designed plan promotes consistent progress and adapts to individual needs, abilities, and goals. In this chapter, we will focus on the fundamental principles of strength training, how to tailor a routine for different fitness levels and ages, and the importance of balancing strength, cardio, and flexibility for optimal health and longevity.

"Through specific, targeted behaviors, you can literally change your destiny by empowering your muscle to run the body's energy-processing and chemical-messaging system in healthy ways." Dr. Gabrielle Lyon

Core Principles of Strength Training: Progressive Overload, Rest, and Recovery

At the heart of effective strength training is the principle of progressive overload—the gradual increase in stress placed on the muscles, which can be achieved by adding weight, increasing repetitions, or incorporating more challenging exercises. Progressive overload stimulates muscle growth, improves strength, and avoids plateaus. Be aware, though, that progressive overload must be approached carefully to prevent injury or burnout.

Equally important are rest and recovery, which are often overlooked. During rest, muscles repair and grow stronger, making it a critical part of training. Overtraining can lead to fatigue, decreased performance, and even injury. Planning ahead, including your rest days, and ensuring sufficient sleep will allow your body to recover and adapt to training stress. Additionally, active recovery activities like yoga, walking, or light stretching can help maintain flexibility and prevent stiffness. Stretching is one of my favorite activities on non-workout days, and my body always thanks me with less stiffness and more energy.

Build an Age-Appropriate Workout Routine for Any Fitness Level

Creating a strength training plan that aligns with your age, fitness level, and goals is important for safety and success. For beginners or older adults, starting with bodyweight exercises, resistance bands, or light weights can build foundational strength without overwhelming the body. Key exercises like squats, lunges, and push-ups can be modified to suit varying abilities. Most gyms offer stationary workout equipment that helps keep it simple, and they have diagrams showing how to perform the entire extension properly. Don't worry about what anyone else is doing or lifting; start where you are and safely build your muscle mass with proper form and sufficient rest.

Intermediate and advanced individuals may combine heavier weights, compound movements (like deadlifts and bench presses), and targeted muscle group training. Regardless of your fitness level, it's vital to prioritize form and technique over intensity to minimize the risk of injury. Training frequency should also reflect individual needs—most people benefit from 2–4 strength sessions per week, depending on their experience and recovery capacity. Take time to regularly assess your progress and adjust your routine to ensure continued growth and adaptability.

Balancing Strength, Cardio, and Flexibility

While strength training is paramount to longevity, it's most effective when combined with cardio and flexibility exercises. Cardiovascular activities like walking, cycling, or swimming improve heart health, lung capacity, and endurance. Including at least 150 minutes of moderate-intensity cardio weekly is recommended for overall health and complements the muscle-strengthening benefits of resistance training. For a well-rounded program, aim for a mix of strength, cardio, and flexibility exercises tailored to individual preferences and goals.

Perfection is not the goal; being consistent is. Customize your routines for your needs and integrate complementary exercises to build a program that promotes lasting strength, health, and vitality. Finding an accountability buddy can make a huge difference. I know it has for me. 90% of the days I did not want to hit the gym, my accountability buddy helped me follow through on my commitment to them and myself. I am always glad afterward, though not always during our workouts.

4

Nutrition for Strength and Longevity

"You can't exercise your way out of a bad diet." Mark Hyman

Nutrition plays a key role in building strength, promoting longevity, and supporting overall health. The foods we consume directly influence muscle growth, recovery, and metabolic efficiency. Let's examine the importance of protein and essential nutrients in muscle development, how your diet can reduce inflammation and support your metabolic health, and discuss strategies for meal timing to optimize performance and recovery.

The Importance of Protein for Muscle Growth and Recovery

How important is protein for muscle growth and repair? Protein is the cornerstone. When you engage in strength training, your muscles experience micro-tears that require amino acids—the building blocks of protein—for repair. Consuming adequate protein ensures your body can rebuild more substantial and resilient muscle tissue. For most people, a daily intake of 0.8–1.2 grams of protein per pound of body weight is optimal, with higher ranges benefiting those engaged in intense training or aging adults combating sarcopenia.

In her book Forever Strong, Dr. Gabrielle Lyon tells us, "Every adult should consume at least 1 gram per pound of their ideal body weight each day. In particular, your first and last meals of the day should each contain a minimum of 30 grams of high-quality protein." We could talk about this topic all day long. Still, to avoid losing focus on the message we are trying to convey in this book. I think the highlight of her comment is "high-quality protein." A Snickers bar may have protein in it, but is that high-quality? Our protein sources are as important as consuming enough protein.

"Animal proteins have around 45% essential amino acids [the ones you have to obtain through diet] whereas plant proteins are between 25 and 35%," per Don Layman, Ph. D. "For example, you need about 2.5 grams of the amino acid leucine to trigger muscle protein synthesis." Animal proteins are naturally higher in leucine, so if you rely on plant sources for protein, you will need to consume more to achieve the long-term results in muscle mass increase. Another thing to consider is that animal proteins are easier to digest. Animal proteins are "about 100% digestible, whereas plant proteins range between 50 and 70% digestible in their natural forms," says Layman. Plant proteins are also high in fiber and are an essential part of our diet.

Beyond protein, other nutrients are equally essential. Healthy fats, particularly omega-3 fatty acids, support joint health and reduce inflammation. Carbohydrates replenish glycogen stores, providing energy for workouts and recovery. Micronutrients like calcium, magnesium, and vitamin D play vital roles in bone health and muscle contraction, while antioxidants from fruits and vegetables help mitigate oxidative stress from exercise. A balanced diet rich in whole foods ensures your body has the tools to build strength and recover effectively.

How Nutrition Supports Metabolic Health and Reduces Inflammation

The right nutrition plan extends its benefits beyond muscle growth and significantly impacts metabolic health. A balanced diet can stabilize blood sugar levels, improve your insulin sensitivity, and support a healthy metabolic rate. For example, high-fiber foods such as whole grains, legumes, and vegetables slow digestion and regulate blood sugar, reducing the risk of insulin resistance—a precursor to type 2 diabetes.

Dr. Casey Means, author of Good Energy, teaches us, "We eat 70 metric tons of food in our lifetimes, and (a) high-quality diet leads to a high-quality life! The answer of "what to eat" is simple: eat real, minimally processed, nutrient-packed food that is grown in the richest, biodiverse soil and ecosystems."We eat food that is grown in the richet, bio

Certain foods have anti-inflammatory properties that combat chronic low-grade inflammation, a key contributor to aging and chronic diseases. Omega-3 fatty acids from fish, nuts, and seeds reduce inflammatory markers, while polyphenols from foods like berries, green tea, and dark chocolate provide additional protective effects. Avoiding processed foods, refined sugars, and trans fats further helps minimize inflammation, creating an environment that facilitates muscle recovery and overall health.

Meal Timing Strategies for Optimizing Performance and Recovery

Timing your meals around workouts can enhance energy levels, improve performance, and accelerate recovery. Consuming a balanced meal 2–3 hours before exercise ensures your body has sufficient fuel to power through training. This pre workout meal should include complex carbohydrates for sustained energy, moderate protein for muscle support, and a small amount of fat for satiety.

After your workout, a post-exercise meal or snack is necessary for recovery. Consuming protein (20–30 grams) within 30–60 minutes of training helps kickstart muscle repair and growth, while carbohydrates replenish depleted glycogen stores. Adding a small amount of healthy fat, such as avocado or nuts, can further support recovery. For those engaging in multiple training sessions or intense workouts, prioritizing quick-digesting carbs like fruits and protein shakes immediately post-workout is incredibly beneficial.

Intermittent fasting or time-restricted eating can also align with strength and longevity goals for some individuals, but care must be taken to ensure adequate nutrient intake during eating windows. Ultimately, the best timing strategy will fit your schedule, support your consistent energy levels, and aid recovery, making your strength training sustainable and effective over the long term.

Nutrition is an integral partner to strength training and longevity. By prioritizing protein, balancing macronutrients, and embracing anti-inflammatory and nutrient-dense foods, you can optimize muscle growth, metabolic health, and recovery.

5

The Mental & Emotional Benefits of Strength Training

Strength training is often celebrated for its physical benefits, but its impact extends much further, by profoundly influencing mental and emotional well-being. Did you know engaging in regular strength training not only reduces stress, anxiety, and depression but also enhances brain health, cognitive function, and emotional resilience. Let's analyze how building physical strength contributes to mental and emotional fortitude, fostering confidence and greater control over life.

A Tool for Reducing Stress, Anxiety, and Depression

Strength training is a powerful stress reliever, offering immediate and long-term benefits. During exercise, your body releases endorphins—neurochemicals that elevate mood and create a sense of well-being. This natural "high" can reduce stress levels and improve emotional outlook. Additionally, strength training lowers cortisol, the body's primary stress hormone, helping to counteract the effects of chronic stress, which can lead to fatigue, irritability, and even physical illness. This is a bonus, epecially for pre or post menopausal women.

"You're only one workout away from a good mood." Kylie Nelson. There is so much truth in this statement.

Regular strength training is linked to significant reductions in anxiety and depression. Studies suggest that resistance exercise alters brain chemistry, by increasing levels of serotonin and dopamine, which are crucial for mood regulation. Strength training offers a structured activity that fosters a sense of accomplishment, helping individuals combat feelings often associated with anxiety and depression. For most of us, completing a challenging workout or lifting weights is a form of active meditation, providing mental clarity and focus.

The Connection Between Exercise, Brain Health, and Cognitive Function

Strength training supports brain health by improving blood flow and stimulating the release of brain-derived neurotrophic factor (BDNF), the protein that promotes the growth and repair of neurons. Higher levels of BDNF are associated with better memory, learning, and overall cognitive function. Research indicates that regular resistance training can slow age-related cognitive decline and reduce the risk of neurodegenerative diseases like Alzheimer's and dementia.

It also enhances executive functions, such as problem-solving, attention, and decision-making, essential for daily life. Exercise-induced improvements in brain health also extend to mental sharpness and creativity. Your brain adapts by engaging the body in physically demanding tasks, strengthening neural pathways, and improving mental agility. Strength training is a great tool for maintaining physical and mental vitality.

Boosting Confidence and Resilience Through Consistent Training

One of the most transformative aspects of strength training is its ability to boost confidence and resilience. Consistent training allows individuals to set and achieve measurable goals, whether that goal is lifting a heavier weight, completing more repetitions, or mastering a new exercise. These accomplishments foster a sense of self-efficacy—the belief in one's ability to overcome challenges—which translates into other areas of life.

Strength training also builds emotional resilience. It takes discipline and perseverance to maintain a consistent training regimen, which can enhance your ability to face adversity and manage stress. The mental toughness developed through regular training creates a foundation of inner strength, empowering individuals to tackle life's challenges with confidence and determination.

"No matter how many mistakes you make or how slow you progress, you are still way ahead of everyone who isn't trying." – Tony Robbins, motivational speaker and fitness advocate.

6

Overcoming Challenges and Staying Motivated

"Start by doing what's necessary, then what's possible; and suddenly you are doing the impossible." -Saint Francis.

Embarking on or continuing a strength training journey can be challenging, especially as we face daily challenges in life, plateaus, or wobbling motivation. The key is persistence and adaptability, recognizing that progress is a marathon, not a sprint. This chapter explores how to start building muscle at any age, strategies for overcoming obstacles, and inspiring success stories of individuals who have transformed their lives and reversed the effects of aging through strength training.

How to Start (or Restart) Building Muscle at Any Age

It's never too late—or too early—to start building muscle. If you are brand new to strength training, your focus should be on mastering the fundamentals: proper form, gradual progression, and consistency. Consulting with a fitness professional or following an age-appropriate program ensures safe and effective progress.

For those restarting after a break, be patient with yourself. Muscle memory will aid in regaining lost strength, but it's essential to gradually ease back into training to avoid overexertion or even injury. Establishing a realistic schedule and tracking progress helps rebuild momentum. Remember, even small steps, like committing to two weekly workouts, can yield significant long-term results. Regardless of age or fitness level, the first step is to start.

Tips for Overcoming Plateaus and Staying Consistent

Plateaus are a normal part of any fitness journey but can be frustrating if not managed. To overcome plateaus, the principle of progressive overload is crucial. Gradually increasing resistance, trying new exercises, or adjusting the number of sets and repetitions can reignite progress. Cross-training—incorporating different forms of exercise like swimming or yoga—can also challenge muscles in new ways and prevent burnout.

Consistency, however, is the cornerstone of long-term success. Building habits around training—such as scheduling workouts at the same time each day or exercising with a partner—helps sustain motivation. Setting clear, attainable goals and celebrating milestones keeps enthusiasm alive. Additionally, varying routines to keep workouts engaging and enjoyable can make strength training feel less like a chore and more like an adventure.

Success Stories of Individuals Who Reversed Aging Through Strength Training

"Success seems to be connected with action. Successful people keep moving. They make mistakes, but they don't quit." -Conrad Hilton.

Real-life success stories are powerful reminders of what's possible through strength training. For example, 70-year-old Joan began strength training after a fall, which left her fearful of losing her independence. Within a year, she regained her confidence, improved her balance, and even participated in her first 5K walk. Her story affirms the life-changing impact of building muscle, even later in life.

Another inspiring example is Carlos, a 55-year-old office worker who struggled with obesity and chronic back pain. After committing to a simple strength training routine, he lost 40 pounds, eliminated his back pain, and reduced his blood pressure to healthy levels. Carlos attributes his renewed energy and outlook on life to the discipline and empowerment he gained through consistent training.

You probably know of one or more people who have this type of success in improving their quality of life with exercise. These stories—and countless others—highlight the potential for strength training to reverse the physical and emotional effects of aging. They prove that with dedication, the right plan, and a supportive mindset, anyone can harness the power of strength to transform their health and vitality.

"Character cannot be developed in ease and quiet. Only through experience of trial and suffering can the soul be strengthened, vision cleared, ambition inspired, and success achieved." Helen Keller, American author

Overcoming challenges and staying motivated in strength training requires persistence, and inspiration. You can do this! By starting at your own pace, finding an accountability partner, embracing consistency, and learning from the successes of others, you can navigate obstacles and stay committed to your journey. Strength training isn't just about building muscle; it's about creating a long life of resilience and health.

7

The Lifestyle of Longevity

Strength training is a cornerstone of longevity, but it's most effective when integrated into a complete approach to health. Achieving vitality and independence at every stage of life requires balancing physical exercise with other essential habits, such as sleep, stress management, hydration, and self-care.

Integrating Strength Training with Other Healthy Habits: Sleep, Stress Management, and Hydration

A longevity-focused lifestyle goes beyond the gym. Quality sleep is foundational; during deep sleep, the body repairs muscles, regulates hormones and consolidates learning. Adults should aim for 7–9 hours of sleep per night (even if it doesn't always happen), creating an environment conducive to rest by limiting screen time, maintaining a consistent bedtime, and managing caffeine intake. We may not always get the sleep we need, especially when raising a family, caring for others, or dealing with day-to-day concerns. It is important to set ourselves up for success by making changes that enable us to improve our sleep whenever possible.

Stress management is equally critical. Chronic stress elevates cortisol levels, hindering muscle recovery, increasing inflammation, and accelerating aging. Incorporating relaxation techniques like meditation, deep breathing, or yoga can help balance the demands of training and daily life. Strength training itself also acts as a stress reliever, promoting mental clarity and emotional resilience.

Another important thing to remember is hydration. It often gets overlooked but is necessary for muscle function and recovery. Water supports nutrient transport, regulates body temperature, and aids joint lubrication. Drinking at least 8–10 glasses of water daily, or more during intense training, can assist you in achieving optimal performance and overall health. Alkaline water is my favorite type; I find it refreshing and free of any aftertaste. By combining these habits with strength training, you can create a synergistic lifestyle that supports longevity.

The Importance of Recovery & Self-Care

"Perseverance is not a long race; it is many short races one after the other." Walter Elliot, former Secretary of State for Scotland

Recovery isn't just a rest period—it's when the body rebuilds and strengthens. Active recovery activities like walking, stretching, or light yoga keep the body moving without placing undue stress on muscles. You may enjoy foam rolling or massage to further support recovery by easing muscle tension and improving circulation.

Self-care also extends to mental and emotional health. Regular check-ins with oneself—whether through journaling, therapy, or mindfulness practices—foster a sense of balance and awareness. Your diet plays a significant role in recovery; eating anti-inflammatory foods like leafy greens, berries, and fatty fish aids muscle repair and reduces oxidative stress. Prioritizing self-care helps sustain the physical and emotional resilience necessary for a longevity-focused lifestyle.

Living a Life of Vitality, Independence, and Strength at Every Stage

Strength training and healthy habits lay the foundation for a vibrant, independent life. Physical strength enhances the ability to easily perform daily activities, while mental resilience allows individuals to approach challenges with confidence and determination. As we age, maintaining vitality becomes less about adding years to life and more about adding life to years.

Living a life of longevity means embracing the journey with purpose. Strength training becomes a lifelong practice, not just a phase, evolving with individual needs and goals. By nurturing a growth mindset and adaptability, individuals can thrive at every stage of life, embodying independence, energy, and strength. The longevity lifestyle is not about avoiding aging but redefining it, proving that vitality is achievable for everyone.

8

Conclusion

Start Your Strength Journey, Today

The path to strength and longevity begins with a single step. Whether you're just starting or reigniting your commitment to health, the path to a stronger, healthier future is always within reach. The science is clear: building and maintaining muscle is one of the most effective ways to extend your vitality, improve your quality of life, and take control of your aging process. Now is the time to take action—your future self will thank you.

Embracing this journey is not about perfection; it's about progress. Each workout, every new skill mastered, and every step taken toward a healthier lifestyle is a victory worth celebrating! Your small, consistent choices today—lifting a weight, trying a new recipe, or prioritizing rest—create the foundation for a stronger tomorrow. Strength training isn't just an activity; it's a process of growth and empowerment that rewards your body and mind alike.

"Energy and persistence conquer all things." Benjamin Franklin, Founding Father of the US

Inspiring Others to Lead Stronger, Longer Lives

Your journey has the power to inspire. Sharing your experiences, challenges, and victories encourages others to prioritize their strength and longevity. Looking and feeling great well into our older years is also a motivating aspect for others that observe our transformation. Leading by example can help create a ripple effect by empowering friends, family, and your community members to embrace healthier, more active lifestyles. Together, we can redefine aging—not as a decline but as an opportunity to grow stronger, more resilient, and more capable.

So, take the leap and begin your ageless strength journey today. Commit to the process, trust in your ability to improve, and celebrate each milestone along the way. The road ahead is filled with possibility, and your dedication to strength will unlock a life of vitality, independence, and joy at every stage. Let's make longevity a movement—one rep, one step, and one life at a time.

Resources

Insurance Services Aiding Pet Owners. https://uberant.com/article/465377-insurance-services-aiding-pet-owners/

Flight Simulator Market Size By 2031 · Bookmark Details. http://www.socialbookmarkssite.com/bookmark/5523222/flight-simulator-market-size-by-2031/

Muscle Loss In Seniors: Can It Be Reversed? - Leading Edge Senior Care. https://leadingedgeseniorcare.com/2024/02/muscle-loss-in-seniors-can-it-be-reversed/

Frontiers | Reference Values for Five-Repetition Chair Stand Test Among Middle-Aged and Elderly Community-Dwelling Chinese Adults. https://www.frontiersin.org/journals/medicine/articles/10.3389/fmed.2021.659107/full

The Importance of Building Muscle Mass and Strength for Weight Loss - Matthew Osborn AEP – Vision Health. https://www.visionexercisephysiology.com.au/the-importance-of-building-muscle-mass-and-strength-for-weight-loss-matthew-osborn-aep/

The Benefits of Strength Training: How it Can Increase Metabolism and Lower Body Fat Percentage | Kaeos Fitness. https://www.kaeosfitness.com/blog/the-benefits-of-strength-training-how-it-can-increase-metabolism-and-lower-body-fat-percentage

(2021). Strategies for strong bones. The Charlotte Post, 47(24), 2B.

Exercise Benefits Beyond the Obvious. https://www.mavfit.com/post/exercise-benefits-beyond-the-obvious

Forever Strong Dr. Gabrielle Lyon

[2]https://drgabriellelyon.com/muscle-centric-medicine/

[3]https://finance.yahoo.com/news/muscle-cornerstone-longevity-140025059.html?guccounter=1

https://www.goodreads.com/work/quotes/124545218-forever-strong-a-new-science-based-strategy-for-aging-well?utm_source=chatgpt.com

Conrad Hilton Quotes and Sayings | Wise Sayings. https://www.wisesayings.com/authors/conrad-hilton-quotes/

The Anti-Aging Benefits of Muscle | Neighborhood Wellness Clinic & Medical Spa. https://neighborhoodwellnessclinic.com/post/the-anti-aging-benefits-of-muscle

Bedtime - ldgslssz.com. https://www.ldgslssz.com/bedtime